Hi I'm Molly,

Over the last 20 years, I've been guiding people through their journey of meal planning and eating healthier. Through those 20 years, I've begun to notice certain trends and patterns that permeate throughout this 'weight-loss' space and I've come to a realization that there is nothing out there that is a 'no-frills' and 'get-to-the-point' sort of resource. Most fad diet books out there promote unhealthy or unsustainable dieting behaviors that can promote harmful food relationships between those wishing to eat healthier. I've written this book to get straight to the point. You will find 30 days' worth of weight-loss, low LDL, and fulfilling healthy recipes that you can repeat year-round. Following this meal plan will give you all the essential nutrients and help you into a calorie deficit. That's guaranteed results from weight loss. Stick with the plan and trust the process. It'll all be worth it!

Let's get straight to it.

Table Of Contents

Day 1:

Breakfast - Avocado and Egg Breakfast Bowl
1/2 avocado, sliced (120 calories)
2 large eggs, scrambled (140 calories)
1 cup spinach, sautéed (7 calories)
1 small tomato, diced (15 calories)
1 slice whole grain toast (80 calories)
Total: 362 calories

Mid-Morning Snack - Greek Yogurt with Berries and Almonds
1/2 cup non-fat Greek yogurt (60 calories)
1/4 cup mixed berries (strawberries, blueberries, raspberries) (20 calories)
1 tablespoon almonds (49 calories)
Total: 129 calories

Lunch - Quinoa and Black Bean Salad
1/2 cup cooked quinoa (111 calories)
1/2 cup black beans, drained and rinsed (110 calories)
1/4 cup corn kernels (30 calories)

1/4 cup diced red bell pepper (10 calories)
2 tablespoons diced red onion (8 calories)
1 tablespoon chopped cilantro (1 calorie)
Juice of 1 lime (10 calories)
Total: 280 calories

Afternoon Snack - Hummus with Carrot Sticks
2 tablespoons hummus (70 calories)
1 cup carrot sticks (52 calories)
Total: 122 calories

Dinner - Grilled Chicken with Sweet Potato and Asparagus
4 oz grilled chicken breast (120 calories)
1 medium sweet potato, baked (103 calories)
1 cup asparagus, grilled or roasted (27 calories)
1 teaspoon olive oil for cooking (40 calories)
Total: 290 calories

Evening Snack - Apple with Peanut Butter
1 medium apple, sliced (95 calories)
1 tablespoon peanut butter (95 calories)

Total: 190 calories

Late-Night Meal - Turkey and Veggie Stir-Fry
4 oz lean ground turkey (120 calories)
1 cup mixed vegetables (broccoli, bell peppers, snap peas) (50 calories)
1 tablespoon low-sodium soy sauce (10 calories)
1/2 tablespoon sesame oil (60 calories)
Total: 240 calories

Daily Total: 1613 calories

Day 2:

Breakfast - Berry Smoothie Bowl
1/2 cup frozen mixed berries (70 calories)
1/2 banana (53 calories)
1/2 cup spinach (3 calories)
1/2 cup unsweetened almond milk (15 calories)
1 tablespoon chia seeds (60 calories)
1 tablespoon honey or maple syrup (60 calories)
Optional toppings: sliced banana, shredded coconut, granola
Total: 261 calories

Mid-Morning Snack - Cottage Cheese with Pineapple
1/2 cup low-fat cottage cheese (80 calories)
1/2 cup diced pineapple (41 calories)
Total: 121 calories

Lunch - Turkey and Avocado Wrap
3 oz sliced turkey breast (90 calories)

1 small whole grain wrap (80 calories)
1/4 avocado, sliced (60 calories)
Lettuce, tomato, cucumber slices
Mustard or Greek yogurt-based dressing
Total: 230 calories

Afternoon Snack - Whole Grain Crackers
with Hummus
6 whole grain crackers (120 calories)
2 tablespoons hummus (70 calories)
Total: 190 calories

Dinner - Baked Salmon with Quinoa and
Steamed Broccoli
4 oz baked salmon fillet (240 calories)
1/2 cup cooked quinoa (111 calories)
Steamed broccoli florets (30 calories)
Lemon wedge for squeezing
Total: 381 calories

Evening Snack - Greek Yogurt with
Almonds and Honey
1/2 cup non-fat Greek yogurt (60 calories)
1 tablespoon slivered almonds (49 calories)

1 teaspoon honey (21 calories)
Total: 130 calories

Late-Night Meal - Veggie Stir-Fry with Tofu
4 oz firm tofu, cubed (94 calories)
1 cup mixed stir-fry vegetables (broccoli,
bell peppers, carrots) (50 calories)
1 tablespoon low-sodium soy sauce (10
calories)
1/2 tablespoon sesame oil (60 calories)
Total: 214 calories
Daily Total: 1527 calories

Day 3:

Breakfast - Veggie Omelette
2 large eggs, beaten (140 calories)
1/4 cup diced bell peppers (10 calories)
1/4 cup diced onions (15 calories)
1/4 cup sliced mushrooms (5 calories)
1 cup spinach (7 calories)
1 teaspoon olive oil for cooking (40 calories)
Total: 217 calories

Mid-Morning Snack - Banana with Almond Butter
1 medium banana (105 calories)
1 tablespoon almond butter (95 calories)
Total: 200 calories

Lunch - Chickpea Salad
1 cup canned chickpeas, drained and rinsed (220 calories)
1/4 cup diced cucumber (4 calories)
1/4 cup diced tomatoes (8 calories)
1/4 cup diced red onion (16 calories)

2 tablespoons chopped parsley (1 calorie)
Juice of 1 lemon (10 calories)
1 tablespoon olive oil (120 calories)
Salt and pepper to taste
Total: 379 calories

Afternoon Snack - Greek Yogurt with Berries
1/2 cup non-fat Greek yogurt (60 calories)
1/4 cup mixed berries (strawberries, blueberries, raspberries) (20 calories)
Total: 80 calories

Dinner - Grilled Chicken Caesar Salad
3 oz grilled chicken breast, sliced (120 calories)
Romaine lettuce (15 calories)
1/4 cup cherry tomatoes (15 calories)
2 tablespoons grated Parmesan cheese (43 calories)
1/4 cup croutons (60 calories)
Caesar dressing (2 tablespoons) (120 calories)
Total: 373 calories

Evening Snack - Cottage Cheese with Pineapple
1/2 cup low-fat cottage cheese (80 calories)
1/2 cup diced pineapple (41 calories)
Total: 121 calories

Late-Night Meal - Turkey and Vegetable Soup
1 cup turkey and vegetable soup (homemade or low-sodium store-bought) (150 calories)
Total: 150 calories
Daily Total: 1520 calories

Day 4:

Breakfast - Blueberry Oatmeal
1/2 cup rolled oats (150 calories)
1 cup unsweetened almond milk (30 calories)
1/4 cup blueberries (21 calories)
1 tablespoon honey or maple syrup (60 calories)
Total: 261 calories

Mid-Morning Snack - Apple Slices with Peanut Butter
1 medium apple (95 calories)
1 tablespoon peanut butter (95 calories)
Total: 190 calories

Lunch - Turkey and Avocado Wrap
3 oz sliced turkey breast (90 calories)
1 small whole grain wrap (80 calories)
1/4 avocado, sliced (60 calories)
Lettuce, tomato, cucumber slices
Mustard or Greek yogurt-based dressing
Total: 230 calories

Afternoon Snack - Greek Yogurt with Almonds
1/2 cup non-fat Greek yogurt (60 calories)
1 tablespoon slivered almonds (49 calories)
Total: 109 calories

Dinner - Baked Salmon with Roasted Vegetables
4 oz baked salmon fillet (240 calories)
1 cup mixed roasted vegetables (zucchini, bell peppers, onions) (100 calories)
Total: 340 calories

Evening Snack - Carrot Sticks with Hummus
1 cup carrot sticks (52 calories)
2 tablespoons hummus (70 calories)
Total: 122 calories

Late-Night Meal - Quinoa Stuffed Bell Peppers
1 bell pepper, halved and deseeded (24 calories)

1/2 cup cooked quinoa (111 calories)
1/4 cup black beans, drained and rinsed (55 calories)
1/4 cup diced tomatoes (8 calories)
1/4 cup shredded cheese (90 calories)
Total: 288 calories

Daily Total: 1540 calories

Day 5:

Breakfast - Spinach and Feta Omelette
2 large eggs, beaten (140 calories)
1/2 cup spinach leaves (3 calories)
2 tablespoons crumbled feta cheese (50 calories)
1 teaspoon olive oil for cooking (40 calories)
Total: 233 calories

Mid-Morning Snack - Banana with Almond Butter
1 medium banana (105 calories)
1 tablespoon almond butter (95 calories)
Total: 200 calories

Lunch - Chicken and Vegetable Stir-Fry
3 oz sliced chicken breast (90 calories)
1 cup mixed stir-fry vegetables (broccoli, bell peppers, snap peas) (50 calories)
1 tablespoon low-sodium soy sauce (10 calories)
1/2 tablespoon sesame oil (60 calories)

Total: 210 calories

Afternoon Snack - Greek Yogurt with
Berries
1/2 cup non-fat Greek yogurt (60 calories)
1/4 cup mixed berries (strawberries,
blueberries, raspberries) (20 calories)
Total: 80 calories

Dinner - Lentil Soup with Whole Grain
Bread
1 cup lentil soup (homemade or low-sodium
store-bought) (150 calories)
1 slice whole grain bread (80 calories)
Total: 230 calories

Evening Snack - Cottage Cheese with
Pineapple
1/2 cup low-fat cottage cheese (80 calories)
1/2 cup diced pineapple (41 calories)
Total: 121 calories

Late-Night Meal - Turkey and Veggie Wrap
3 oz sliced turkey breast (90 calories)

1 small whole grain wrap (80 calories)
Lettuce, tomato, cucumber slices
Mustard or Greek yogurt-based dressing
Total: 170 calories

Daily Total: 1324 calories

Day 6:

Breakfast - Banana Peanut Butter Smoothie
1 medium banana (105 calories)
1 tablespoon peanut butter (95 calories)
1 cup unsweetened almond milk (30
calories)
1 tablespoon honey or maple syrup (60
calories)
Total: 290 calories

Mid-Morning Snack - Apple Slices with
Almond Butter
1 medium apple (95 calories)
1 tablespoon almond butter (95 calories)
Total: 190 calories

Lunch - Chickpea Salad
1 cup canned chickpeas, drained and rinsed
(220 calories)
1/4 cup diced cucumber (4 calories)
1/4 cup diced tomatoes (8 calories)
1/4 cup diced red onion (16 calories)

2 tablespoons chopped parsley (1 calorie)
Juice of 1 lemon (10 calories)
1 tablespoon olive oil (120 calories)
Salt and pepper to taste
Total: 379 calories

Afternoon Snack - Greek Yogurt with Almonds
1/2 cup non-fat Greek yogurt (60 calories)
1 tablespoon slivered almonds (49 calories)
Total: 109 calories

Dinner - Grilled Chicken with Sweet Potato Mash and Steamed Green Beans
4 oz grilled chicken breast (120 calories)
1 medium sweet potato, mashed (103 calories)
1 cup steamed green beans (44 calories)
Total: 267 calories

Evening Snack - Carrot Sticks with Hummus
1 cup carrot sticks (52 calories)
2 tablespoons hummus (70 calories)

Total: 122 calories

Late-Night Meal - Quinoa Salad with Veggies
1/2 cup cooked quinoa (111 calories)
1/4 cup diced bell peppers (10 calories)
1/4 cup diced cucumber (4 calories)
1/4 cup cherry tomatoes, halved (9 calories)
1 tablespoon chopped parsley (1 calorie)
Juice of 1 lemon (10 calories)
1 tablespoon olive oil (120 calories)
Total: 265 calories

Daily Total: 1422 calories

Day 7:

Breakfast - Greek Yogurt Parfait
1/2 cup non-fat Greek yogurt (60 calories)
1/4 cup granola (120 calories)
1/4 cup mixed berries (strawberries,
blueberries, raspberries) (20 calories)
Total: 200 calories

Mid-Morning Snack - Whole Grain
Crackers with Hummus
6 whole grain crackers (120 calories)
2 tablespoons hummus (70 calories)
Total: 190 calories

Lunch - Tuna Salad Wrap
1/2 cup canned tuna in water, drained (120
calories)
1 small whole grain wrap (80 calories)
1/4 cup diced celery (4 calories)
1/4 cup diced red onion (16 calories)
2 tablespoons plain Greek yogurt (15
calories)

Lettuce, tomato
Total: 235 calories

Afternoon Snack - Apple Slices with Peanut
Butter
1 medium apple (95 calories)
1 tablespoon peanut butter (95 calories)
Total: 190 calories

Dinner - Beef and Vegetable Stir-Fry
3 oz sliced beef sirloin (180 calories)
1 cup mixed stir-fry vegetables (broccoli,
bell peppers, snap peas) (50 calories)
1 tablespoon low-sodium soy sauce (10
calories)
1/2 tablespoon sesame oil (60 calories)
Total: 300 calories

Evening Snack - Cottage Cheese with
Pineapple
1/2 cup low-fat cottage cheese (80 calories)
1/2 cup diced pineapple (41 calories)
Total: 121 calories

Late-Night Meal - Veggie and Bean Soup
1 cup vegetable and bean soup (homemade
or low-sodium store-bought) (150 calories)
Total: 150 calories

Daily Total: 1376 calories

Day 8:

Breakfast - Scrambled Eggs with Spinach and Feta
2 large eggs, scrambled (140 calories)
1/2 cup spinach, sautéed (3 calories)
2 tablespoons crumbled feta cheese (50 calories)
Total: 193 calories

Mid-Morning Snack - Greek Yogurt with Berries
1/2 cup non-fat Greek yogurt (60 calories)
1/4 cup mixed berries (strawberries, blueberries, raspberries) (20 calories)
Total: 80 calories

Lunch - Grilled Veggie and Hummus Wrap
1 small whole grain wrap (80 calories)
2 tablespoons hummus (70 calories)
Grilled vegetables (zucchini, bell peppers, eggplant) (50 calories)
Total: 200 calories

Afternoon Snack - Carrot Sticks with Guacamole
1 cup carrot sticks (52 calories)
2 tablespoons guacamole (60 calories)
Total: 112 calories

Dinner - Baked Chicken with Roasted Sweet Potatoes and Green Beans
4 oz baked chicken breast (120 calories)
1 medium sweet potato, roasted (103 calories)
1 cup steamed green beans (44 calories)
Total: 267 calories

Evening Snack - Cottage Cheese with Pineapple
1/2 cup low-fat cottage cheese (80 calories)
1/2 cup diced pineapple (41 calories)
Total: 121 calories

Late-Night Meal - Turkey and Black Bean Chili

1 cup turkey and black bean chili
(homemade or low-sodium store-bought)
(200 calories)
Total: 200 calories

Daily Total: 1233 calories

Day 9:

Breakfast - Banana Walnut Overnight Oats
1/2 cup rolled oats (150 calories)
1/2 cup unsweetened almond milk (15 calories)
1/2 banana, mashed (53 calories)
1 tablespoon chopped walnuts (52 calories)
1 tablespoon honey or maple syrup (60 calories)
Total: 330 calories

Mid-Morning Snack - Apple Slices with Almond Butter
1 medium apple (95 calories)
1 tablespoon almond butter (95 calories)
Total: 190 calories

Lunch - Chickpea and Avocado Salad
1 cup canned chickpeas, drained and rinsed (220 calories)
1/4 avocado, diced (60 calories)
1/4 cup diced cucumber (4 calories)

1/4 cup diced tomatoes (8 calories)
2 tablespoons chopped parsley (1 calorie)
Juice of 1 lemon (10 calories)
1 tablespoon olive oil (120 calories)
Total: 423 calories

Afternoon Snack - Greek Yogurt with Almonds
1/2 cup non-fat Greek yogurt (60 calories)
1 tablespoon slivered almonds (49 calories)
Total: 109 calories

Dinner - Grilled Salmon with Quinoa and Steamed Broccoli
4 oz grilled salmon fillet (240 calories)
1/2 cup cooked quinoa (111 calories)
1 cup steamed broccoli (55 calories)
Total: 406 calories

Evening Snack - Carrot Sticks with Hummus
1 cup carrot sticks (52 calories)
2 tablespoons hummus (70 calories)
Total: 122 calories

Late-Night Meal - Lentil and Vegetable Soup
1 cup lentil and vegetable soup (homemade or low-sodium store-bought) (150 calories)
Total: 150 calories

Daily Total: 1730 calories

Day 10:

Breakfast - Veggie and Cheese Omelette
2 large eggs, beaten (140 calories)
1/4 cup diced bell peppers (10 calories)
1/4 cup diced onions (15 calories)
1/4 cup diced tomatoes (8 calories)
2 tablespoons shredded cheese (80 calories)
Total: 253 calories

Mid-Morning Snack - Greek Yogurt with
Berries
1/2 cup non-fat Greek yogurt (60 calories)
1/4 cup mixed berries (strawberries,
blueberries, raspberries) (20 calories)
Total: 80 calories

Lunch - Turkey and Avocado Wrap
3 oz sliced turkey breast (90 calories)
1 small whole grain wrap (80 calories)
1/4 avocado, sliced (60 calories)
Lettuce, tomato, cucumber slices
Mustard or Greek yogurt-based dressing

Total: 230 calories

Afternoon Snack - Whole Grain Crackers
with Hummus
6 whole grain crackers (120 calories)
2 tablespoons hummus (70 calories)
Total: 190 calories

Dinner - Grilled Chicken with Quinoa Salad
4 oz grilled chicken breast (120 calories)
1/2 cup cooked quinoa (111 calories)
Mixed greens, cherry tomatoes, cucumber,
red onion
Balsamic vinaigrette dressing (1 tablespoon)
(50 calories)
Total: 281 calories

Evening Snack - Cottage Cheese with
Pineapple
1/2 cup low-fat cottage cheese (80 calories)
1/2 cup diced pineapple (41 calories)
Total: 121 calories

Late-Night Meal - Vegetarian Stir-Fry with Tofu
1 cup mixed stir-fry vegetables (broccoli, bell peppers, snap peas) (50 calories)
4 oz firm tofu, cubed (94 calories)
1 tablespoon low-sodium soy sauce (10 calories)
1/2 tablespoon sesame oil (60 calories)
Total: 214 calories

Daily Total: 1369 calories

Day 11:

Breakfast - Blueberry Protein Pancakes
2 whole grain pancakes (200 calories)
1/2 cup fresh blueberries (42 calories)
1 tablespoon maple syrup (52 calories)
Total: 294 calories

Mid-Morning Snack - Apple Slices with Peanut Butter
1 medium apple (95 calories)
1 tablespoon peanut butter (95 calories)
Total: 190 calories

Lunch - Quinoa and Black Bean Salad
1/2 cup cooked quinoa (111 calories)
1/2 cup black beans, drained and rinsed (110 calories)
1/4 cup corn kernels (30 calories)
1/4 cup diced red bell pepper (10 calories)
2 tablespoons diced red onion (8 calories)
1 tablespoon chopped cilantro (1 calorie)
Juice of 1 lime (10 calories)

Total: 280 calories

Afternoon Snack - Greek Yogurt with Almonds
1/2 cup non-fat Greek yogurt (60 calories)
1 tablespoon slivered almonds (49 calories)
Total: 109 calories

Dinner - Baked Salmon with Roasted Vegetables
4 oz baked salmon fillet (240 calories)
1 cup mixed roasted vegetables (zucchini, bell peppers, onions) (100 calories)
Total: 340 calories

Evening Snack - Carrot Sticks with Hummus
1 cup carrot sticks (52 calories)
2 tablespoons hummus (70 calories)
Total: 122 calories

Late-Night Meal - Lentil Soup with Whole Grain Bread

1 cup lentil soup (homemade or low-sodium store-bought) (150 calories)
1 slice whole grain bread (80 calories)
Total: 230 calories

Daily Total: 1565 calories

Day 12:

Breakfast - Greek Yogurt Parfait
1/2 cup non-fat Greek yogurt (60 calories)
1/4 cup granola (120 calories)
1/4 cup mixed berries (strawberries,
blueberries, raspberries) (20 calories)
Total: 200 calories

Mid-Morning Snack - Cottage Cheese with
Pineapple
1/2 cup low-fat cottage cheese (80 calories)
1/2 cup diced pineapple (41 calories)
Total: 121 calories

Lunch - Turkey and Veggie Wrap
3 oz sliced turkey breast (90 calories)
1 small whole grain wrap (80 calories)
Lettuce, tomato, cucumber slices
Mustard or Greek yogurt-based dressing
Total: 170 calories

Afternoon Snack - Apple Slices with Almond Butter
1 medium apple (95 calories)
1 tablespoon almond butter (95 calories)
Total: 190 calories

Dinner - Grilled Chicken with Quinoa and Steamed Broccoli
4 oz grilled chicken breast (120 calories)
1/2 cup cooked quinoa (111 calories)
1 cup steamed broccoli (55 calories)
Total: 286 calories

Evening Snack - Carrot Sticks with Hummus
1 cup carrot sticks (52 calories)
2 tablespoons hummus (70 calories)
Total: 122 calories

Late-Night Meal - Lentil Soup with Whole Grain Bread
1 cup lentil soup (homemade or low-sodium store-bought) (150 calories)
1 slice whole grain bread (80 calories)

Total: 230 calories

Daily Total: 1319 calories

Day 13:

Breakfast - Avocado Toast
1 slice whole grain bread (80 calories)
1/4 avocado, mashed (60 calories)
Sliced tomato and cucumber (20 calories)
Sprinkle of salt and pepper
Total: 160 calories

Mid-Morning Snack - Banana with Peanut Butter
1 medium banana (105 calories)
1 tablespoon peanut butter (95 calories)
Total: 200 calories

Lunch - Grilled Chicken Salad
3 oz grilled chicken breast, sliced (120 calories)
Mixed greens (lettuce, spinach, arugula) (15 calories)
Cherry tomatoes, sliced (15 calories)
1/4 cup sliced cucumber (4 calories)
1/4 cup sliced bell peppers (10 calories)

Balsamic vinaigrette dressing (1 tbsp) (50 calories)
Total: 214 calories

Afternoon Snack - Greek Yogurt with Berries and Almonds
1/2 cup non-fat Greek yogurt (60 calories)
1/4 cup mixed berries (strawberries, blueberries, raspberries) (20 calories)
1 tablespoon almonds (49 calories)
Total: 129 calories

Dinner - Baked Salmon with Quinoa and Steamed Broccoli
4 oz baked salmon fillet (240 calories)
1/2 cup cooked quinoa (111 calories)
Steamed broccoli florets (30 calories)
Lemon wedge for squeezing
Total: 381 calories

Evening Snack - Cottage Cheese with Pineapple
1/2 cup low-fat cottage cheese (80 calories)
1/2 cup diced pineapple (41 calories)

Total: 121 calories

Late-Night Meal - Veggie Stir-Fry with Tofu
1 cup mixed stir-fry vegetables (broccoli,
bell peppers, snap peas) (50 calories)
4 oz firm tofu, cubed (94 calories)
1 tablespoon low-sodium soy sauce (10
calories)
1/2 tablespoon sesame oil (60 calories)
Total: 214 calories

Daily Total: 1419 calories

Day 14:

Breakfast - Berry Smoothie Bowl
1/2 cup frozen mixed berries (70 calories)
1/2 banana (53 calories)
1/2 cup spinach (3 calories)
1/2 cup unsweetened almond milk (15 calories)
1 tablespoon chia seeds (60 calories)
1 tablespoon honey or maple syrup (60 calories)
Optional toppings: sliced banana, shredded coconut, granola
Total: 261 calories

Mid-Morning Snack - Greek Yogurt with Berries and Almonds
1/2 cup non-fat Greek yogurt (60 calories)
1/4 cup mixed berries (strawberries, blueberries, raspberries) (20 calories)
1 tablespoon almonds (49 calories)
Total: 129 calories

Lunch - Quinoa and Black Bean Salad
1/2 cup cooked quinoa (111 calories)
1/2 cup black beans, drained and rinsed (110 calories)
1/4 cup corn kernels (30 calories)
1/4 cup diced red bell pepper (10 calories)
2 tablespoons diced red onion (8 calories)
1 tablespoon chopped cilantro (1 calorie)
Juice of 1 lime (10 calories)
Total: 280 calories

Afternoon Snack - Hummus with Carrot Sticks
2 tablespoons hummus (70 calories)
1 cup carrot sticks (52 calories)
Total: 122 calories

Dinner - Grilled Chicken with Sweet Potato and Asparagus
4 oz grilled chicken breast (120 calories)
1 medium sweet potato, baked (103 calories)
1 cup asparagus, grilled or roasted (27 calories)
1 teaspoon olive oil for cooking (40 calories)

Total: 290 calories

Evening Snack - Greek Yogurt with
Almonds and Honey
1/2 cup non-fat Greek yogurt (60 calories)
1 tablespoon slivered almonds (49 calories)
1 teaspoon honey (21 calories)
Total: 130 calories

Late-Night Meal - Turkey and Vegetable
Soup
1 cup turkey and vegetable soup (homemade
or low-sodium store-bought) (150 calories)
Total: 150 calories

Day 15:

Breakfast - Veggie Omelette
2 large eggs, beaten (140 calories)
1/4 cup diced bell peppers (10 calories)
1/4 cup diced onions (15 calories)
1/4 cup diced tomatoes (8 calories)
1/2 cup spinach (7 calories)
1 teaspoon olive oil for cooking (40 calories)
Total: 220 calories

Mid-Morning Snack - Greek Yogurt with Berries
1/2 cup non-fat Greek yogurt (60 calories)
1/4 cup mixed berries (strawberries, blueberries, raspberries) (20 calories)
Total: 80 calories

Lunch - Turkey and Avocado Wrap
3 oz sliced turkey breast (90 calories)
1 small whole grain wrap (80 calories)
1/4 avocado, sliced (60 calories)
Lettuce, tomato, cucumber slices

Mustard or Greek yogurt-based dressing
Total: 230 calories

Afternoon Snack - Apple Slices with Peanut
Butter
1 medium apple (95 calories)
1 tablespoon peanut butter (95 calories)
Total: 190 calories

Dinner - Baked Salmon with Roasted
Vegetables
4 oz baked salmon fillet (240 calories)
1 cup mixed roasted vegetables (zucchini,
bell peppers, onions) (100 calories)
Total: 340 calories

Evening Snack - Carrot Sticks with
Hummus
1 cup carrot sticks (52 calories)
2 tablespoons hummus (70 calories)
Total: 122 calories

Late-Night Meal - Lentil Soup with Whole
Grain Bread

1 cup lentil soup (homemade or low-sodium store-bought) (150 calories)
1 slice whole grain bread (80 calories)
Total: 230 calories

Daily Total: 1432 calories

Day 16:

Breakfast - Banana Walnut Overnight Oats
1/2 cup rolled oats (150 calories)
1/2 cup unsweetened almond milk (15 calories)
1/2 banana, mashed (53 calories)
1 tablespoon chopped walnuts (52 calories)
1 tablespoon honey or maple syrup (60 calories)
Total: 330 calories

Mid-Morning Snack - Apple Slices with Almond Butter
1 medium apple (95 calories)
1 tablespoon almond butter (95 calories)
Total: 190 calories

Lunch - Chickpea and Avocado Salad
1 cup canned chickpeas, drained and rinsed (220 calories)
1/4 avocado, diced (60 calories)
1/4 cup diced cucumber (4 calories)

1/4 cup diced tomatoes (8 calories)
2 tablespoons chopped parsley (1 calorie)
Juice of 1 lemon (10 calories)
1 tablespoon olive oil (120 calories)
Total: 423 calories

Afternoon Snack - Greek Yogurt with Almonds
1/2 cup non-fat Greek yogurt (60 calories)
1 tablespoon slivered almonds (49 calories)
Total: 109 calories

Dinner - Grilled Chicken with Quinoa and Steamed Broccoli
4 oz grilled chicken breast (120 calories)
1/2 cup cooked quinoa (111 calories)
1 cup steamed broccoli (55 calories)
Total: 286 calories

Evening Snack - Cottage Cheese with Pineapple
1/2 cup low-fat cottage cheese (80 calories)
1/2 cup diced pineapple (41 calories)
Total: 121 calories

Late-Night Meal - Veggie Stir-Fry with Tofu
1 cup mixed stir-fry vegetables (broccoli,
bell peppers, snap peas) (50 calories)
4 oz firm tofu, cubed (94 calories)
1 tablespoon low-sodium soy sauce (10
calories)
1/2 tablespoon sesame oil (60 calories)
Total: 214 calories

Daily Total: 1673 calories

Day 17:

Breakfast - Blueberry Protein Pancakes
2 whole grain pancakes (200 calories)
1/2 cup fresh blueberries (42 calories)
1 tablespoon maple syrup (52 calories)
Total: 294 calories

Mid-Morning Snack - Apple Slices with
Peanut Butter
1 medium apple (95 calories)
1 tablespoon peanut butter (95 calories)
Total: 190 calories

Lunch - Quinoa and Black Bean Salad
1/2 cup cooked quinoa (111 calories)
1/2 cup black beans, drained and rinsed (110
calories)
1/4 cup corn kernels (30 calories)
1/4 cup diced red bell pepper (10 calories)
2 tablespoons diced red onion (8 calories)
1 tablespoon chopped cilantro (1 calorie)
Juice of 1 lime (10 calories)

Total: 280 calories

Afternoon Snack - Hummus with Carrot Sticks
2 tablespoons hummus (70 calories)
1 cup carrot sticks (52 calories)
Total: 122 calories

Dinner - Grilled Chicken with Sweet Potato and Asparagus
4 oz grilled chicken breast (120 calories)
1 medium sweet potato, baked (103 calories)
1 cup asparagus, grilled or roasted (27 calories)
1 teaspoon olive oil for cooking (40 calories)
Total: 290 calories

Evening Snack - Greek Yogurt with Almonds and Honey
1/2 cup non-fat Greek yogurt (60 calories)
1 tablespoon slivered almonds (49 calories)
1 teaspoon honey (21 calories)
Total: 130 calories

Late-Night Meal - Turkey and Vegetable Soup
1 cup turkey and vegetable soup (homemade or low-sodium store-bought) (150 calories)
Total: 150 calories

Daily Total: 1366 calories

Day 18:

Breakfast - Veggie Omelette
2 large eggs, beaten (140 calories)
1/4 cup diced bell peppers (10 calories)
1/4 cup diced onions (15 calories)
1/4 cup diced tomatoes (8 calories)
1/2 cup spinach (7 calories)
1 teaspoon olive oil for cooking (40 calories)
Total: 220 calories

Mid-Morning Snack - Greek Yogurt with Berries
1/2 cup non-fat Greek yogurt (60 calories)
1/4 cup mixed berries (strawberries, blueberries, raspberries) (20 calories)
Total: 80 calories

Lunch - Turkey and Avocado Wrap
3 oz sliced turkey breast (90 calories)
1 small whole grain wrap (80 calories)
1/4 avocado, sliced (60 calories)
Lettuce, tomato, cucumber slices

Mustard or Greek yogurt-based dressing
Total: 230 calories

Afternoon Snack - Apple Slices with Peanut
Butter
1 medium apple (95 calories)
1 tablespoon peanut butter (95 calories)
Total: 190 calories

Dinner - Baked Salmon with Roasted
Vegetables
4 oz baked salmon fillet (240 calories)
1 cup mixed roasted vegetables (zucchini,
bell peppers, onions) (100 calories)
Total: 340 calories

Evening Snack - Carrot Sticks with
Hummus
1 cup carrot sticks (52 calories)
2 tablespoons hummus (70 calories)
Total: 122 calories

Late-Night Meal - Lentil Soup with Whole
Grain Bread

1 cup lentil soup (homemade or low-sodium store-bought) (150 calories)
1 slice whole grain bread (80 calories)
Total: 230 calories

Daily Total: 1432 calories

Day 19:

Breakfast - Banana Walnut Overnight Oats
1/2 cup rolled oats (150 calories)
1/2 cup unsweetened almond milk (15 calories)
1/2 banana, mashed (53 calories)
1 tablespoon chopped walnuts (52 calories)
1 tablespoon honey or maple syrup (60 calories)
Total: 330 calories

Mid-Morning Snack - Apple Slices with Almond Butter
1 medium apple (95 calories)
1 tablespoon almond butter (95 calories)
Total: 190 calories

Lunch - Chickpea and Avocado Salad
1 cup canned chickpeas, drained and rinsed (220 calories)
1/4 avocado, diced (60 calories)
1/4 cup diced cucumber (4 calories)

1/4 cup diced tomatoes (8 calories)
2 tablespoons chopped parsley (1 calorie)
Juice of 1 lemon (10 calories)
1 tablespoon olive oil (120 calories)
Total: 423 calories

Afternoon Snack - Greek Yogurt with Almonds
1/2 cup non-fat Greek yogurt (60 calories)
1 tablespoon slivered almonds (49 calories)
Total: 109 calories

Dinner - Grilled Chicken with Quinoa and Steamed Broccoli
4 oz grilled chicken breast (120 calories)
1/2 cup cooked quinoa (111 calories)
1 cup steamed broccoli (55 calories)
Total: 286 calories

Evening Snack - Cottage Cheese with Pineapple
1/2 cup low-fat cottage cheese (80 calories)
1/2 cup diced pineapple (41 calories)
Total: 121 calories

Late-Night Meal - Veggie Stir-Fry with Tofu
1 cup mixed stir-fry vegetables (broccoli,
bell peppers, snap peas) (50 calories)
4 oz firm tofu, cubed (94 calories)
1 tablespoon low-sodium soy sauce (10
calories)
1/2 tablespoon sesame oil (60 calories)
Total: 214 calories

Daily Total: 1673 calories

Day 20:

Breakfast - Blueberry Protein Pancakes
2 whole grain pancakes (200 calories)
1/2 cup fresh blueberries (42 calories)
1 tablespoon maple syrup (52 calories)
Total: 294 calories

Mid-Morning Snack - Apple Slices with
Peanut Butter
1 medium apple (95 calories)
1 tablespoon peanut butter (95 calories)
Total: 190 calories

Lunch - Quinoa and Black Bean Salad
1/2 cup cooked quinoa (111 calories)
1/2 cup black beans, drained and rinsed (110
calories)
1/4 cup corn kernels (30 calories)
1/4 cup diced red bell pepper (10 calories)
2 tablespoons diced red onion (8 calories)
1 tablespoon chopped cilantro (1 calorie)
Juice of 1 lime (10 calories)

Total: 280 calories

Afternoon Snack - Hummus with Carrot Sticks
2 tablespoons hummus (70 calories)
1 cup carrot sticks (52 calories)
Total: 122 calories

Dinner - Grilled Chicken with Sweet Potato and Asparagus
4 oz grilled chicken breast (120 calories)
1 medium sweet potato, baked (103 calories)
1 cup asparagus, grilled or roasted (27 calories)
1 teaspoon olive oil for cooking (40 calories)
Total: 290 calories

Evening Snack - Greek Yogurt with Almonds and Honey
1/2 cup non-fat Greek yogurt (60 calories)
1 tablespoon slivered almonds (49 calories)
1 teaspoon honey (21 calories)
Total: 130 calories

Late-Night Meal - Turkey and Vegetable
Soup
1 cup turkey and vegetable soup (homemade
or low-sodium store-bought) (150 calories)
Total: 150 calories

Daily Total: 1456 calories

Day 21:

Breakfast - Veggie Omelette
2 large eggs, beaten (140 calories)
1/4 cup diced bell peppers (10 calories)
1/4 cup diced onions (15 calories)
1/4 cup diced tomatoes (8 calories)
1/2 cup spinach (7 calories)
1 teaspoon olive oil for cooking (40 calories)
Total: 220 calories

Mid-Morning Snack - Greek Yogurt with Berries
1/2 cup non-fat Greek yogurt (60 calories)
1/4 cup mixed berries (strawberries, blueberries, raspberries) (20 calories)
Total: 80 calories

Lunch - Turkey and Avocado Wrap
3 oz sliced turkey breast (90 calories)
1 small whole grain wrap (80 calories)
1/4 avocado, sliced (60 calories)
Lettuce, tomato, cucumber slices

Mustard or Greek yogurt-based dressing
Total: 230 calories

Afternoon Snack - Apple Slices with Peanut
Butter
1 medium apple (95 calories)
1 tablespoon peanut butter (95 calories)
Total: 190 calories

Dinner - Baked Salmon with Roasted
Vegetables
4 oz baked salmon fillet (240 calories)
1 cup mixed roasted vegetables (zucchini,
bell peppers, onions) (100 calories)
Total: 340 calories

Evening Snack - Carrot Sticks with
Hummus
1 cup carrot sticks (52 calories)
2 tablespoons hummus (70 calories)
Total: 122 calories

Late-Night Meal - Lentil Soup with Whole
Grain Bread

1 cup lentil soup (homemade or low-sodium store-bought) (150 calories)
1 slice whole grain bread (80 calories)
Total: 230 calories

Daily Total: 1232 calories

Day 22:

Breakfast - Banana Walnut Overnight Oats
1/2 cup rolled oats (150 calories)
1/2 cup unsweetened almond milk (15 calories)
1/2 banana, mashed (53 calories)
1 tablespoon chopped walnuts (52 calories)
1 tablespoon honey or maple syrup (60 calories)
Total: 330 calories

Mid-Morning Snack - Apple Slices with Almond Butter
1 medium apple (95 calories)
1 tablespoon almond butter (95 calories)
Total: 190 calories

Lunch - Chickpea and Avocado Salad
1 cup canned chickpeas, drained and rinsed (220 calories)
1/4 avocado, diced (60 calories)
1/4 cup diced cucumber (4 calories)

1/4 cup diced tomatoes (8 calories)
2 tablespoons chopped parsley (1 calorie)
Juice of 1 lemon (10 calories)
1 tablespoon olive oil (120 calories)
Total: 423 calories

Afternoon Snack - Greek Yogurt with Almonds
1/2 cup non-fat Greek yogurt (60 calories)
1 tablespoon slivered almonds (49 calories)
Total: 109 calories

Dinner - Grilled Chicken with Quinoa and Steamed Broccoli
4 oz grilled chicken breast (120 calories)
1/2 cup cooked quinoa (111 calories)
1 cup steamed broccoli (55 calories)
Total: 286 calories

Evening Snack - Cottage Cheese with Pineapple
1/2 cup low-fat cottage cheese (80 calories)
1/2 cup diced pineapple (41 calories)
Total: 121 calories

Late-Night Meal - Veggie Stir-Fry with Tofu
1 cup mixed stir-fry vegetables (broccoli,
bell peppers, snap peas) (50 calories)
4 oz firm tofu, cubed (94 calories)
1 tablespoon low-sodium soy sauce (10
calories)
1/2 tablespoon sesame oil (60 calories)
Total: 214 calories

Daily Total: 1673 calories

Day 23:

Breakfast - Blueberry Protein Pancakes
2 whole grain pancakes (200 calories)
1/2 cup fresh blueberries (42 calories)
1 tablespoon maple syrup (52 calories)
Total: 294 calories

Mid-Morning Snack - Apple Slices with Peanut Butter
1 medium apple (95 calories)
1 tablespoon peanut butter (95 calories)
Total: 190 calories

Lunch - Quinoa and Black Bean Salad
1/2 cup cooked quinoa (111 calories)
1/2 cup black beans, drained and rinsed (110 calories)
1/4 cup corn kernels (30 calories)
1/4 cup diced red bell pepper (10 calories)
2 tablespoons diced red onion (8 calories)
1 tablespoon chopped cilantro (1 calorie)
Juice of 1 lime (10 calories)

Total: 280 calories

Afternoon Snack - Hummus with Carrot
Sticks
2 tablespoons hummus (70 calories)
1 cup carrot sticks (52 calories)
Total: 122 calories

Dinner - Grilled Chicken with Sweet Potato
and Asparagus
4 oz grilled chicken breast (120 calories)
1 medium sweet potato, baked (103 calories)
1 cup asparagus, grilled or roasted (27
calories)
1 teaspoon olive oil for cooking (40 calories)
Total: 290 calories

Evening Snack - Greek Yogurt with
Almonds and Honey
1/2 cup non-fat Greek yogurt (60 calories)
1 tablespoon slivered almonds (49 calories)
1 teaspoon honey (21 calories)
Total: 130 calories

Late-Night Meal - Turkey and Vegetable Soup

1 cup turkey and vegetable soup (homemade or low-sodium store-bought) (150 calories)
Total: 150 calories

Daily Total: 1456 calories

Day 24:

Breakfast - Veggie Omelette
2 large eggs, beaten (140 calories)
1/4 cup diced bell peppers (10 calories)
1/4 cup diced onions (15 calories)
1/4 cup diced tomatoes (8 calories)
1/2 cup spinach (7 calories)
1 teaspoon olive oil for cooking (40 calories)
Total: 220 calories

Mid-Morning Snack - Greek Yogurt with Berries
1/2 cup non-fat Greek yogurt (60 calories)
1/4 cup mixed berries (strawberries, blueberries, raspberries) (20 calories)
Total: 80 calories

Lunch - Turkey and Avocado Wrap
3 oz sliced turkey breast (90 calories)
1 small whole grain wrap (80 calories)
1/4 avocado, sliced (60 calories)
Lettuce, tomato, cucumber slices

Mustard or Greek yogurt-based dressing
Total: 230 calories

Afternoon Snack - Apple Slices with Peanut
Butter
1 medium apple (95 calories)
1 tablespoon peanut butter (95 calories)
Total: 190 calories

Dinner - Baked Salmon with Roasted
Vegetables
4 oz baked salmon fillet (240 calories)
1 cup mixed roasted vegetables (zucchini,
bell peppers, onions) (100 calories)
Total: 340 calories

Evening Snack - Carrot Sticks with
Hummus
1 cup carrot sticks (52 calories)
2 tablespoons hummus (70 calories)
Total: 122 calories

Late-Night Meal - Lentil Soup with Whole
Grain Bread

1 cup lentil soup (homemade or low-sodium store-bought) (150 calories)
1 slice whole grain bread (80 calories)
Total: 230 calories

Daily Total: 1432 calories

Day 25:

Breakfast - Banana Walnut Overnight Oats
1/2 cup rolled oats (150 calories)
1/2 cup unsweetened almond milk (15 calories)
1/2 banana, mashed (53 calories)
1 tablespoon chopped walnuts (52 calories)
1 tablespoon honey or maple syrup (60 calories)
Total: 330 calories

Mid-Morning Snack - Apple Slices with Almond Butter
1 medium apple (95 calories)
1 tablespoon almond butter (95 calories)
Total: 190 calories

Lunch - Chickpea and Avocado Salad
1 cup canned chickpeas, drained and rinsed (220 calories)
1/4 avocado, diced (60 calories)
1/4 cup diced cucumber (4 calories)

1/4 cup diced tomatoes (8 calories)
2 tablespoons chopped parsley (1 calorie)
Juice of 1 lemon (10 calories)
1 tablespoon olive oil (120 calories)
Total: 423 calories

Afternoon Snack - Greek Yogurt with Almonds
1/2 cup non-fat Greek yogurt (60 calories)
1 tablespoon slivered almonds (49 calories)
Total: 109 calories

Dinner - Grilled Chicken with Quinoa and Steamed Broccoli
4 oz grilled chicken breast (120 calories)
1/2 cup cooked quinoa (111 calories)
1 cup steamed broccoli (55 calories)
Total: 286 calories

Evening Snack - Cottage Cheese with Pineapple
1/2 cup low-fat cottage cheese (80 calories)
1/2 cup diced pineapple (41 calories)
Total: 121 calories

Late-Night Meal - Veggie Stir-Fry with Tofu
1 cup mixed stir-fry vegetables (broccoli,
bell peppers, snap peas) (50 calories)
4 oz firm tofu, cubed (94 calories)
1 tablespoon low-sodium soy sauce (10
calories)
1/2 tablespoon sesame oil (60 calories)
Total: 214 calories

Daily Total: 1673 calories

Day 26:

Breakfast - Blueberry Protein Pancakes
2 whole grain pancakes (200 calories)
1/2 cup fresh blueberries (42 calories)
1 tablespoon maple syrup (52 calories)
Total: 294 calories

Mid-Morning Snack - Apple Slices with Peanut Butter
1 medium apple (95 calories)
1 tablespoon peanut butter (95 calories)
Total: 190 calories

Lunch - Quinoa and Black Bean Salad
1/2 cup cooked quinoa (111 calories)
1/2 cup black beans, drained and rinsed (110 calories)
1/4 cup corn kernels (30 calories)
1/4 cup diced red bell pepper (10 calories)
2 tablespoons diced red onion (8 calories)
1 tablespoon chopped cilantro (1 calorie)
Juice of 1 lime (10 calories)

Total: 280 calories

Afternoon Snack - Hummus with Carrot
Sticks
2 tablespoons hummus (70 calories)
1 cup carrot sticks (52 calories)
Total: 122 calories

Dinner - Grilled Chicken with Sweet Potato
and Asparagus
4 oz grilled chicken breast (120 calories)
1 medium sweet potato, baked (103 calories)
1 cup asparagus, grilled or roasted (27
calories)
1 teaspoon olive oil for cooking (40 calories)
Total: 290 calories

Evening Snack - Greek Yogurt with
Almonds and Honey
1/2 cup non-fat Greek yogurt (60 calories)
1 tablespoon slivered almonds (49 calories)
1 teaspoon honey (21 calories)
Total: 130 calories

Late-Night Meal - Turkey and Vegetable
Soup
1 cup turkey and vegetable soup (homemade
or low-sodium store-bought) (150 calories)
Total: 150 calories

Daily Total: 1456 calories

Day 27:

Breakfast - Veggie Omelette
2 large eggs, beaten (140 calories)
1/4 cup diced bell peppers (10 calories)
1/4 cup diced onions (15 calories)
1/4 cup diced tomatoes (8 calories)
1/2 cup spinach (7 calories)
1 teaspoon olive oil for cooking (40 calories)
Total: 220 calories

Mid-Morning Snack - Greek Yogurt with Berries
1/2 cup non-fat Greek yogurt (60 calories)
1/4 cup mixed berries (strawberries, blueberries, raspberries) (20 calories)
Total: 80 calories

Lunch - Turkey and Avocado Wrap
3 oz sliced turkey breast (90 calories)
1 small whole grain wrap (80 calories)
1/4 avocado, sliced (60 calories)
Lettuce, tomato, cucumber slices

Mustard or Greek yogurt-based dressing
Total: 230 calories

Afternoon Snack - Apple Slices with Peanut
Butter
1 medium apple (95 calories)
1 tablespoon peanut butter (95 calories)
Total: 190 calories

Dinner - Baked Salmon with Roasted
Vegetables
4 oz baked salmon fillet (240 calories)
1 cup mixed roasted vegetables (zucchini,
bell peppers, onions) (100 calories)
Total: 340 calories

Evening Snack - Carrot Sticks with
Hummus
1 cup carrot sticks (52 calories)
2 tablespoons hummus (70 calories)
Total: 122 calories

Late-Night Meal - Lentil Soup with Whole
Grain Bread

1 cup lentil soup (homemade or low-sodium store-bought) (150 calories)
1 slice whole grain bread (80 calories)
Total: 230 calories

Daily Total: 1432 calories

Day 28:

Breakfast - Banana Walnut Overnight Oats
1/2 cup rolled oats (150 calories)
1/2 cup unsweetened almond milk (15 calories)
1/2 banana, mashed (53 calories)
1 tablespoon chopped walnuts (52 calories)
1 tablespoon honey or maple syrup (60 calories)
Total: 330 calories

Mid-Morning Snack - Apple Slices with Almond Butter
1 medium apple (95 calories)
1 tablespoon almond butter (95 calories)
Total: 190 calories

Lunch - Chickpea and Avocado Salad
1 cup canned chickpeas, drained and rinsed (220 calories)
1/4 avocado, diced (60 calories)
1/4 cup diced cucumber (4 calories)

1/4 cup diced tomatoes (8 calories)
2 tablespoons chopped parsley (1 calorie)
Juice of 1 lemon (10 calories)
1 tablespoon olive oil (120 calories)
Total: 423 calories

Afternoon Snack - Greek Yogurt with Almonds
1/2 cup non-fat Greek yogurt (60 calories)
1 tablespoon slivered almonds (49 calories)
Total: 109 calories

Dinner - Grilled Chicken with Quinoa and Steamed Broccoli
4 oz grilled chicken breast (120 calories)
1/2 cup cooked quinoa (111 calories)
1 cup steamed broccoli (55 calories)
Total: 286 calories

Evening Snack - Cottage Cheese with Pineapple
1/2 cup low-fat cottage cheese (80 calories)
1/2 cup diced pineapple (41 calories)
Total: 121 calories

Late-Night Meal - Veggie Stir-Fry with Tofu
1 cup mixed stir-fry vegetables (broccoli,
bell peppers, snap peas) (50 calories)
4 oz firm tofu, cubed (94 calories)
1 tablespoon low-sodium soy sauce (10
calories)
1/2 tablespoon sesame oil (60 calories)
Total: 214 calories
Daily Total: 1673 calories

Day 29:

Breakfast - Blueberry Protein Pancakes
2 whole grain pancakes (200 calories)
1/2 cup fresh blueberries (42 calories)
1 tablespoon maple syrup (52 calories)
Total: 294 calories

Mid-Morning Snack - Apple Slices with Peanut Butter
1 medium apple (95 calories)
1 tablespoon peanut butter (95 calories)
Total: 190 calories

Lunch - Quinoa and Black Bean Salad
1/2 cup cooked quinoa (111 calories)
1/2 cup black beans, drained and rinsed (110 calories)
1/4 cup corn kernels (30 calories)
1/4 cup diced red bell pepper (10 calories)
2 tablespoons diced red onion (8 calories)
1 tablespoon chopped cilantro (1 calorie)
Juice of 1 lime (10 calories)

Total: 280 calories

Afternoon Snack - Hummus with Carrot
Sticks
2 tablespoons hummus (70 calories)
1 cup carrot sticks (52 calories)
Total: 122 calories

Dinner - Grilled Chicken with Sweet Potato
and Asparagus
4 oz grilled chicken breast (120 calories)
1 medium sweet potato, baked (103 calories)
1 cup asparagus, grilled or roasted (27
calories)
1 teaspoon olive oil for cooking (40 calories)
Total: 290 calories

Evening Snack - Greek Yogurt with
Almonds and Honey
1/2 cup non-fat Greek yogurt (60 calories)
1 tablespoon slivered almonds (49 calories)
1 teaspoon honey (21 calories)
Total: 130 calories

Late-Night Meal - Turkey and Vegetable
Soup
1 cup turkey and vegetable soup (homemade
or low-sodium store-bought) (150 calories)
Total: 150 calories
Daily Total: 1456 calories

Day 30:

Breakfast - Veggie Omelette
2 large eggs, beaten (140 calories)
1/4 cup diced bell peppers (10 calories)
1/4 cup diced onions (15 calories)
1/4 cup diced tomatoes (8 calories)
1/2 cup spinach (7 calories)
1 teaspoon olive oil for cooking (40 calories)
Total: 220 calories

Mid-Morning Snack - Greek Yogurt with Berries
1/2 cup non-fat Greek yogurt (60 calories)
1/4 cup mixed berries (strawberries, blueberries, raspberries) (20 calories)
Total: 80 calories

Lunch - Turkey and Avocado Wrap
3 oz sliced turkey breast (90 calories)
1 small whole grain wrap (80 calories)
1/4 avocado, sliced (60 calories)
Lettuce, tomato, cucumber slices

Mustard or Greek yogurt-based dressing
Total: 230 calories

Afternoon Snack - Apple Slices with Peanut
Butter
1 medium apple (95 calories)
1 tablespoon peanut butter (95 calories)
Total: 190 calories

Dinner - Baked Salmon with Roasted
Vegetables
4 oz baked salmon fillet (240 calories)
1 cup mixed roasted vegetables (zucchini,
bell peppers, onions) (100 calories)
Total: 340 calories

Evening Snack - Carrot Sticks with
Hummus
1 cup carrot sticks (52 calories)
2 tablespoons hummus (70 calories)
Total: 122 calories

Late-Night Meal - Lentil Soup with Whole
Grain Bread

1 cup lentil soup (homemade or low-sodium store-bought) (150 calories)
1 slice whole grain bread (80 calories)
Total: 230 calories
Daily Total: 1432 calories